Energetic Equipoise

Mindfulness in Sports Performance

Table of Contents

Chapter 1. Introduction

Discover the dynamic balance between physical prowess and mental fortitude in our Special Report titled "Energetic Equipoise: Mindfulness in Sports Performance". This illuminating resource delves into the world of sports, where athletes not only unleash their body's potential but also tap into the power of their minds. Through vivid, captivating narration and real-world examples, we unravel the significance of mindfulness and its consequential impact on an athlete's peak performance. This engaging and relatable report is designed to inspire athletes, coaches, and sports enthusiasts alike, blending cutting-edge research with practical, actionable tactics. Use this valuable guide to unlock a new level of performance, fostering a harmonious balance between body and mind. Get ready to transform your understanding of sports performance - because the game isn't just played in the stadium, it's played in the mind too. Secure your copy today and embark on an exciting journey toward achieving energetic equipoise.

Chapter 2. The Intersection of Mindfulness and Physical Activity

The exploration of mindfulness within the realm of physical training asks us to reassess and redefine prevailing notions of strength, endurance, and performance. Traditional thinking persuades us to consider these traits as purely physical in nature - a simplistic understanding that fails to conceive sports performance as a holistic process. With advancements in modern research, the importance of the mind in optimizing sports performance has been recognized. Consequently, the role of mindfulness becomes vital to consider within the context of physical activity.

2.1. The Significance of Mindfulness

Mindfulness, to define it in a comprehensive manner, constitutes a state of conscious awareness wherein an individual is truly present in each moment. This involves a profound attention to and awareness of one's emotions, thoughts, and sensations in relation to his or her surroundings. People practicing mindfulness are capable of recognizing their mental and physical states without becoming overly reactive. Unsurprisingly, these principles of acceptance, concentration, and non-judgment can have transformative impacts on a sportsperson's performance.

One-dimensional models of training that focus solely on physical enhancement risk neglecting the mental stamina athletes need for achieving peak performance. Competitive sporting environments are often nerve-wracking, stressful, and emotionally demanding. The ability to manage these challenges and maintain composure is often the difference between good and great. The practice of mindfulness offers a powerful tool for athletes to cultivate this mental fortitude.

By remaining mindful, sportspersons can keep their concentration grounded in the present, thus allowing them to react effectively to any competitive situation.

2.2. The Confluence of Mindfulness and Physical Training

The intersection of mindfulness and physical activity can be understood through the concept of flow, a state of heightened focus and immersion in activities such as sports. Hungarian psychologist Mihaly Csikszentmihalyi, who conceptualized this term, described flow as a state wherein individuals are so involved in an activity that nothing else seems to matter. This scenario is all too familiar for athletes who describe similar experiences of being "in the zone". In these instances, their execution feels effortless, precise, and controlled.

Integrating mindfulness within physical training can facilitate athletes' access to this state of flow. By enhancing their awareness and concentration, mindfulness practices help sportspeople remain focused on the task at hand, boosting their likelihood of achieving this coveted and performance-enhancing state of flow.

2.3. Mindfulness-Based Activities and Improved Athletic Performance

Mindfulness-based practices, such as meditation and yoga, can serve as standalone exercises or complementary additions to traditional training regimens. With the aim of promoting mental well-being and resilience, they offer multiple advantages to athletes. Research has revealed links between these practices and increased concentration, improved reaction times, lower stress levels, and a higher degree of control over emotional responses. All these elements proceeding benefits embodied better sports performance.

In the world of professional sports, many successful athletes have openly recognized the pivotal role of mindfulness in their training. NBA player LeBron James, for example, has publicly expressed his use of mindfulness practices, which he credits for helping maintain his composure during high-pressure games. In the realm of tennis, superstar Novak Djokovic endorses mindful meditation as a core element of his training, equating mental strength to enduring success.

2.4. The Intersection: A Practical Perspective

From a practical perspective, incorporating mindfulness into physical activities isn't as complex as it may seem. It involves promoting an awareness of one's physical sensations, cognitions, and emotions during training and performance. This could be as simple as focusing on one's breathing during a cool-down session, or taking a moment to center oneself before a big game.

Mindfulness exercises can be seamlessly woven into an athlete's daily routine; a powerful tool for becoming attuned to their bodies and nurturing resilience in difficulty. Furthermore, mindfulness can be used as a relational tool, helping athletes form healthier interactions within their team or with their opponents - a crucial aspect often overlooked in traditional competitive sporting narratives.

The correlation of mindfulness and physical activity epitomizes the foundation of our discussions on 'Energetic Equipoise'. Far from being unrelated domains, the mental and physical aspects of sports performance are intrinsically linked, each fueling the other. As we continue to explore this connection, our holistic perspective on sports performance evolves - an evolution that holds the promise of unimagined potential and extraordinary human achievement for athletes, coaches, and sports enthusiasts worldwide.

By embracing mindfulness, athletes of all levels can transcend barriers, reaching new heights of performance by establishing a captivating harmony between mind and body. The presence of mindfulness in physical activity is now impossible to disregard. As we step into an age where holistic perspectives are replacing outdated mind-body dichotomies, the path to achieving energetic equipoise in sports performance becomes increasingly clear.

Chapter 3. Decoding the Athlete's Mindset: An Exploration

The mind of an athlete, much like the physical attributes, is conditioned and cultivated over time. It isn't a product of simple genetics or dumb luck, but rather the cumulative result of preparation, discipline, and a deep internal drive to excel. This chapter intends to explore and unpack the mindset of elite athletes, cast in light of the scientific research in sports psychology, neuroscience, and related fields.

3.1. Embracing the Success and Failure Spectrum

At the heart of an athlete's mindset is the understanding that success and failure are not binary but, instead, two sides of the same coin. An athlete perceives failure not as an end but as an essential, potentially rewarding step towards success. This resilience to adversity is fueled by an intrinsic motivation and a committed work ethic.

This comprehension expands the athlete's bandwidth for resilience, transforming setbacks into learning opportunities. Embracing failure teaches athletes to manage discomfort, boosting their tolerance in high-pressure environments. The outcome is a mind primed for performance, mastering the art of handling both triumph and disappointment with equal grace.

3.2. The Concept of Grit

Angela Duckworth, in her seminal work "Grit: The Power of Passion and Perseverance", postulates that the long-term commitment to individual goals, or grit, is a more substantial predictor of success than innate talent. Grit abounds in the elite athletic mindset, serving as a psychological backbone that supports, propels, and sustains performance.

Duckworth's 'Grit Scale' tries to quantify this trait, parsing through factors like follow-through, interest consistency, and the significance of setbacks. Critical to the concept of grit is the notion that hard work, coupled with relentless focus, supersedes inborn aptitude in reaching one's potential. Athletes, in their journey of repetitive training and performance enhancement, embody this tenet wholeheartedly.

3.3. The Power of Visualization

One of the most pervasive tools in an athlete's mental arsenal is visualization or mental imagery. Visualization allows athletes to rehearse their performance in their mind's eye, serving as a catalyst for both physical preparation and mental readiness.

Numerous studies in neuroscience reveal that the act of visualizing an action activates the same brain areas as physically performing the action. Visualization effectively provides an additional practice avenue, contributing to performance improvement. Athletes leverage this mental conditioning to navigate potential challenges, strategize optimal responses, and reinforce a positive, performance-oriented outlook.

3.4. Mindful Athletes: Presence Over Pressure

Today's best athletes do not just train their bodies; they train their minds to stay present. Mindfulness, or the capacity to be fully present and engaged in the here and now, forms the cornerstone of such mental training. Mindful athletes employ various practices, including meditation and breath-work, to foster focus, resilience, and equanimity, all of which contribute significantly to exemplary performance.

Jon Kabat-Zinn, the pioneer of mindfulness-based stress reduction, characterizes mindfulness as "(paying) attention in a particular way; on purpose, in the present moment, and nonjudgmentally." This mindful presence strips away distractions, allowing athletes to compete without the burden of past failures or future anxieties, ultimately improving their performance.

3.5. The Self-Talk Paradigm

Internal dialogues or self-talk emerge as pivotal components in an athlete's psychological toolkit. Meta-analytic reviews and experimental studies have identified self-talk as an efficacious strategy for enhancing athletic performance, demonstrating its influence on attention, motivation, and self-efficacy.

Both instructional and motivational self-talk have proven beneficial. Instructional self-talk helps refine technique and coordination, while motivational self-tal increases endurance and strength. The intentional cultivation of positive self-dialogues, therefore, can play crucial roles in shaping an athlete's mindset and accomplishments.

3.6. Reflection: The Athlete's Mirror

For athletes, reflection—the intentional contemplation and analysis of experiences—provides an essential mechanism for learning and progress. By reflecting on their practice sessions or games, athletes gain insights into their performances, identify weaknesses or errors, and devise strategies to overcome them.

A reflective mindset embraces a no-blame culture, viewing mistakes as opportunities rather than failures. Through reflection, athletes develop a higher sense of self-awareness, empowering them to control their performance and progress.

3.7. Emotional Intelligence: The Unseen Advantage

The ability to identify, understand, and manage emotions—known as emotional intelligence—holds substantial predictive power for the athlete's performance. High emotional intelligence allows athletes to remain mentally tough and composed during high-stress moments, manage their own and others' emotions efficiently, and maintain constructive interpersonal relationships within the team. Consequently, emotional intelligence can be considered an unseen advantage, an edge that allows athletes to thrive.

In conclusion, the athletic mindset is a finely tuned combination of grit, resilience, mindfulness, reflective thinking, and emotional intelligence. Athletes aren't simply born great—they cultivate greatness over time. This exploration underlines the importance of mental strength as an integral part of athletic success, illustrating how the marriage of physical prowess and mental fortitude redefines the playing field. Just as athletes tirelessly work on their physical skills, so too must they exercise their mental muscles to support and enhance their performance. The mind, as any athlete will tell you, is the most potent tool in their arsenal.

Chapter 4. The Science Behind Sports Performance: A Deeper Understanding

Every athletic performance emerges from a complex interplay of physical achievements and mental strengths. This intricate dance involves a diverse expanse of systems within the human body and mind, from the microscopic level of cells and neurotransmitters, towards the macro level of muscles and motions. The endeavor of athletic achievement demands a robust understanding of these systems and an exploration into creating equilibrium.

4.1. The Anatomy of Physical Performance

Understanding sports performance unveils the extensive orchestration between numerous body systems. Muscular strength stands as one of the most recognizable components. The transformation of a puny, underused bicep into a rock-solid muscle occurs through the process of muscle hypertrophy. As we stress our muscles with weighted resistance, tiny muscle fibers undergo trauma, leading to protein synthesis to repair, enlarge, and strengthen these fibers.

Yet, muscles don't move independently; the skeletal system offers them levers and support. Studies show that weight-bearing exercises can stimulate new bone growth, leading to enhanced strength and injury prevention. Meanwhile, tendons and ligaments provide another crucial aspect of the structure, with exercises that encourage flexibility and minimize injury on this front.

Next, we pivot towards the cardiovascular system. A sprinter's fast-twitch muscle fibers get their much-needed oxygen from the cardiovascular system, while distance runners might attribute their endurance to expertly conditioned heart and lung muscles pumping oxygen effectively.

Diet and nutrition also play an integral role in fueling these systems. A balanced diet high in protein aids muscle growth; complex carbohydrates provide sustained energy, and vitamins, minerals, and antioxidants contribute to overall health and recovery. However, the importance of rest and recovery should not be underestimated, as it enables the body to heal, build more robust muscles, and consolidate neuro-muscular memory of the techniques practiced.

4.2. Mental Mastery: The Cognitive Side of Sports Performance

While physical training hones an athlete's body, sports psychology aims to sharpen their mind. Mental strength forms a paramount pillar in achieving peak performance, often serving as the determining factor between equally skilled competitors.

One key aspect of mental prowess in sports is focus. Athletes work relentlessly to filter out distractions and maintain a laser-like concentration on their goals. They cultivate the ability to redirect their focus rapidly in response to changing situations during a match or race. The importance of this skill is evidenced in research; studies indicate that elite athletes often demonstrate superior focus skills compared to non-athletes.

Another mental factor is motivation. It can be internal, originating from the athlete's drive to succeed, or external, linked to rewards or recognition. Regardless of the source, motivation fuels continuous effort, pushing athletes to perform their best and transcend their limitations.

Moreover, athletes exhibit a high degree of mental resilience and tenacity. The ability to bounce back after a loss, cope with injury, or endure grueling training schedules is often embedded in an athlete's mindset. Mental resilience is intertwined with optimism and a strong sense of self-belief, both powerful antibodies against adversity.

Cognitive functions like decision-making and planning also take center stage, especially in team sports. Athletes continually make split-second decisions, calculate risk and reward, and plan their strategies. A sharpened cognitive ability bolsters these skills, translating to stellar on-field performances.

Mindfulness and relaxation techniques like meditation can enhance these mental aspects, leading to lower stress, improved focus, and robust mental health. The result is a mentally conditioned athlete, ready to rise to the challenges of their sporting journey.

4.3. Integrating Physical and Mental Realms for Optimal Performance

Energetic equipoise is not an isolated goal but an evolving process, a dance where the physical and mental entities continuously readjust to maintain balance. Sports performance, seen through this prism, no longer remains a series of disconnected occurrences.

For instance, physical training can shape mental attributes. The discipline, resilience, and concentration required to stick to a rigorous physical training regimen could enhance an athlete's mental fortitude. On the other hand, mental strategies can bolster physical performance. Visualization techniques could improve technical skills, while stress management could enhance recovery and physical health.

Moreover, the fusion of mind and body extends beyond training. Proper nutrition can impact one's mood and cognition, sleep can determine motivation levels, and a positive mindset can influence injury recovery. Therefore, holistic approaches often yield the most compelling results.

In conclusion, the science behind sports performance uncovers a vibrant, dynamic world where body and mind intertwine in a delicate balance. The pursuit of athletic excellence pivots on understanding this intricate relationship and nurturing it systematically. With awareness and practice, energetic equipoise can take sports performance from good to startlingly great. Explore more in our following chapters as we dive into practical strategies, real-world examples of their application, and possible future directions for this exciting field.

Chapter 5. Frameworks for Achieving Energetic Equipoise

Energetic equipoise is at the heart of every breakthrough athletic performance. At first glance, it may appear that the path to such balance is paved solely by physical conditioning. However, crucial yet often overlooked elements in an athlete's training regime are mental fortitude and mindfulness. This dynamic duo sets the foundation for a holistic approach to sports performance that propels athletes from good to exceptional.

5.1. The Dichotomy of Mental Fortitude and Physical Prowess

On one hand, we have physical prowess—an athlete's body conditioned to the pinnacle of fitness, capable of executing phenomenal feats of strength, speed, and stamina. On the other hand, we have mental fortitude—a resilient mindset that perseveres through adversities, harnesses focus, and cultivates a winning spirit. The union of physical prowess and mental fortitude don't just coexist; they interact, intermingle, and intersect in an intricate dance, contributing to overall sports performance. They form the two sides of the same coin, neither more important than the other, both critical to the pursuit of peak performance.

5.2. Digging Deeper: The Concept of Mindfulness

An essential aspect of mental fortitude is mindfulness. Often associated with meditation, the application of mindfulness in sports extends way beyond the yoga mat. To put it simply, mindfulness is a state of present-moment awareness. When athletes are in this state, they're completely tuned into their bodies, the environment, and the task at hand. They remain hyper-focused and unperturbed by distractions or stressors. The magic of mindfulness occurs when this state promotes maximum engagement with training and performance, leading to superior results.

5.3. Mindfulness, Physical Prowess, and Energetic Equipoise

Mindfulness has a symbiotic relationship with physical prowess. By enhancing focus, mindfulness allows athletes to connect deeply with their bodies, amplifying physical prowess. They become more aware of their posture, movement, and breathing, leading to more fluid actions, graceful agility, and improved stamina. This interconnectedness sets the stage for energetic equipoise. When mental attentiveness supports peak physical performance, it not only leads to better results but also promotes an intrinsic sense of well-being and fulfillment.

5.4. Implementing Mindfulness: Practical Tactics

While the concept may seem abstract, incorporating mindfulness into athletic practice is simpler than it might first appear. Deep breathing exercises, body scans, visualization, and even simple mantra repetition are all effective techniques. Athletes can also utilize yoga and meditation as complementary practices, fostering mindfulness both on and off the field. The key to success lies in consistency—rather than an occasional effort, mindfulness should be an integral, daily part of an athlete's routine.

5.5. Embodying Energetic Equipoise: Case Studies

The world of sports is filled with examples where mindfulness and mental fortitude have propelled athletes towards greatness. Top performers like Kobe Bryant, Michael Jordan, Serena Williams, Kerri Walsh Jennings, and Novak Djokovic have all spoken on record about the vital role that mental strength and mindfulness played in their careers. By studying these athletes, insights can be gleaned into how they harnessed the power of their minds, providing a roadmap for other athletes aiming to cultivate their inner equilibrium.

5.6. Assessing Progress: Indicators of Energetic Equipoise

Evaluating the attainment of energetic equipoise is crucial for an athlete's continuous improvement. Tangible indicators such as improved performance, lower stress levels, enhanced focus during high-pressure situations, and rebounding quickly from setbacks can signal progress. Regular self-reflection, seeking feedback, and using mental training logs also offer valuable data for ongoing refinement of mindfulness practices.

The journey towards energetic equipoise may be rigorous, but it can be the distinguishing factor that propels athletes from merely good to extraordinary. Much more than the heat of competition, athletic performance is a holistic blend of physical prowess, mental fortitude, and mindfulness. Achieving this equilibrium does more than elevate the game—it can transform an individual's relationship with sports, unlocking a whole new level of fulfillment and passion.

Through the insights presented here, athletes, coaches, and sports enthusiasts can gain a deeper understanding of how to tap into this powerful resource. Energetic equipoise may well be the unseen advantage that is waiting to transform your life in sports. Embrace it, and watch how it sparks a transformation, not only in the stadium but also in the powerful landscape of the mind.

Chapter 6. Case Studies: Mindfulness in Action

As we progress deeper into the realm of mindfulness in sports, let's focus our attention on real-world examples where this dynamic blend of mental and physical prowess is at its zenith. These case studies offer compelling insights into the lives of athletes who've harnessed the power of mindfulness to reach their peak.

6.1. The Michael Jordan Phenomenon

No discussion of mindfulness in sports can be complete without mentioning basketball legend Michael Jordan. Known for his intense focus on the court, Jordan often described himself in a "zone" during games. His unwavering concentration, a clear manifestation of mindfulness, allowed him to navigate the chaotic court calmly and make critical decisions in mere seconds, often outperforming his competitors.

- **The Mindful Free-throw Technique**: The free-throw line, often described as the loneliest place in basketball, showcases an athlete's mental strength. Jordan would often state that he would envision the ball going through the hoop even before taking the shot, a prime example of visualization, a critical component of mindfulness practice.

6.2. Emulating Eckhart: Chess Grandmaster Magnus Carlsen

Ask anyone who plays chess, and they'll tell you it's much more a mental game than a physical one. Magnus Carlsen, the reigning Chess

World Champion, has often spoken about the influence of Eckhart Tolle's teachings on his play. Tolle's mindfulness-based approach has helped him build mental fortitude and resilience.

- **Power of Now**: Carlsen implements Tolle's 'Power of Now' concept into his gameplay by immersing himself fully in the current move, undistracted by what has transpired previously or what is yet to come. This laser focus enables him to perform under high-pressure situations, a testament to mental solidity developed through mindfulness.

6.3. Carla Suarez Navarro: Conquering Battles On and Off the Field

Spanish professional tennis player Carla Suarez Navarro openly battled Hodgkin Lymphoma while maintaining an impressive presence in the sports world. The mental tenacity found in Suarez Navarro's story provides significant evidence for mindfulness's role in sports.

- **Mindful Healing**: Mindfulness was integral to Suarez Navarro's recovery, often participating in mindfulness-based stress reduction (MBSR) therapy. Her mindfulness practice helped mitigate stress and enhance her overall mental resilience, contributing significantly to her fight against a life-threatening illness while maintaining competitive performance levels.

6.4. The Atlanta Falcons: The Team that Breathes Together wins Together

American football team the Atlanta Falcons incorporated mindfulness and yoga into their training regime. The 2016 Super Bowl finalists bear testimony to the power of mindfulness in team sports, resulting in improved team cohesion and individual performance.

- **Group Mindfulness Practice**: Players engage in group mindfulness practices, synchronized breathing activities that foster a sense of unity and cohesion. This shared experience is said to enhance team spirit and focus on winning collectively, cementing the power of mindfulness on team performance.

6.5. Unraveling the "Djoker": Novak Djokovic

The tennis juggernaut Novak Djokovic owes much of his success to a devoted mindfulness and meditation regime. His ability to remain calm under pressure is a direct result of everyday commitment to mindfulness training.

- **Rituals and Routines**: Djokovic is known for his pre-match routines that include a combination of breathing exercises, dynamic meditation, and tactical visualization. These rituals help him to get into the 'zone,' regulate his emotions, stay focused, and perform under pressure.

While each of these case studies is unique, they carry a shared thread - the recognition of the power of mindfulness and the impact it can have on performance. As each athlete has shown, there is as much a

mental game to play as there is a physical one. Through mindfulness, they have maximized their potential and redefined what it means to be an athlete, all by achieving an energetic equipoise. Their stories serve as useful touchstones for anyone seeking to imbue their sports performance with mindfulness. Their success drives us to ask not whether we should adopt mindfulness, but rather, how soon can we incorporate it into our lives.

Chapter 7. Developing Mental Resilience Within the Sporting Arena

Sporting excellence is not confined solely to the realm of physical prowess. While physical skills are visible and well recognized, an essential, albeit often overlooked factor contributing to peak performance is a robust mental framework. This aspect, encompassed by mental resilience, plays an indispensable part in differentiating a good athlete from a truly great one.

7.1. The Concept of Mental Resilience

Mental resilience refers to an individual's capacity to endure stress, adversity, and bouncing back stronger than before. Undeniably, sports performance, with its potent cocktail of pressure, competition, and unpredictability, is often a breeding ground for mental toughness to thrive.

But what does it mean to possess mental resilience in the sporting context? It isn't just about coping with defeat or managing stress. Instead, it's a multifaceted concept incorporating self-confidence, motivation, concentration, and the capacity to regulate emotions.

7.2. Building Blocks of Mental Resilience

Medical and sports literature have identified several key components that contribute to mental resilience. These elements can serve as a useful framework for understanding and enhancing mental resilience in athletes.

1. Self-belief: An unshakeable belief in one's ability drives athletes to push their limits. This does not ignore failures and setbacks but treats them as stepping stones to eventual success.

2. Motivation: An intrinsic drive fuels the passion to persevere despite challenges. It enables athletes to remain dedicated and focused on their objectives regardless of circumstances.

3. Control: Athletes with mental resilience sense control over their performance and destiny. They feel that their hard work and strategies significantly impact their ultimate success, instead of it being hostage to external factors.

4. Emotional Regulation: This refers to the ability to handle high-pressure situations without succumbing to panic or fear. Individuals who manage their emotions skillfully are less likely to crumble under pressure.

7.3. Developing Mental Resilience: An Overview

A common misconception is that mental resilience is an inherent trait, something you're either born with or without. However, research affirms that like physical strength, mental resilience too can be cultivated and reinforced through deliberate practice and training.

7.4. Fostering Self-Belief

Pouring faith into your own skills, even in the face of adversities, is an essential quality of a mentally resilient athlete. This can be cultivated through reflective practices such as journaling, where athletes can review their successes and identify their strengths. Affirmation exercises can further reinforce this self-belief, where athletes regularly iterate positive beliefs about their capabilities and potential.

7.5. Fueling Intrinsic Motivation

Intrinsic motivation acts as a lasting spark in an athlete's journey, driving them to push their boundaries and persist despite setbacks. Coaches and mentors play a pivotal role in fueling this motivation. This can include setting challenging yet achievable goals, creating supportive environments that foster curiosity and enjoyment, and providing constructive feedback to guide the athlete's progress.

7.6. Embracing Control

Upon understanding that hard work and their strategies significantly impact their success, athletes can focus intensively on elements within their control. This could include training schedules, dietary habits, rest routines, or specific skills. Recognizing what they can control can also help athletes let go of factors beyond their grasp, reducing the stress associated with them.

7.7. Enhancing Emotional Regulation

Training in emotional regulation often involves techniques from fields like cognitive-behavioral therapy and mindfulness. This can involve practices like progressive muscle relaxation (PMR), visualization, and biofeedback. These techniques can help athletes remain calm under pressure, manage their arousal levels, and channel their focus effectively.

7.8. The Role of Coaches in Building Mental Resilience

Coaches, owing to their influential role in an athlete's development, carry a significant responsibility for fostering mental resilience. This can involve setting the right expectations, cultivating a growth mindset, providing challenging yet achievable goals, and encouraging athletes to step out of their comfort zone. Coaches also need to emphasize the importance of mental strength and resilience just as much as, if not more than, physical fitness.

7.9. Mental Resilience and Burnout

A particularly significant aspect of mental resilience in sports is its role in preventing burnout. Athletes, particularly at high-performance levels, often struggle with high levels of stress, which can lead to exhaustion, reduced interest, and often, burnouts. Cultivating mental resilience can equip athletes with coping mechanisms needed to manage this stress, thereby reducing the risk of burnout.

In conclusion, developing mental strength and resilience is as crucial to an athlete's performance as their physical training. Its components - including self-belief, motivation, emotional control, and control - can be purposefully trained to enhance an athlete's performance and longevity in the sports arena. By fostering these qualities, athletes can not only excel in their chosen sport but also apply these principles to other facets of life to maintain overall wellbeing and success, long after they've left the sporting arena.

Chapter 8. Mind-Body Training Regimens for Peak Performance

The world of sports often empowers athletes to train their bodies intensively, pushing their physical limits to reach remarkable athletic feats. Rarely, though, is commemorated the parallel training that thrives within the invisible walls of an athlete's mind. The discipline required to endure discomfort, focus, decision making, and emotional control are nothing short of mental Olympiads. Achieving equipoise between the mind and body that results in peak performance necessitates specific regimens and practices. Let's delve into this path that unifies the mind and body, optimizing athletes to perform at their best.

8.1. Mindfulness and its Interplay with Athletic Performance

Mindfulness, a psychological process involving attention and acceptance, can be a highly effective tool athletes can employ. Attention refers to being tuned in and aware of the current experience, both internally and externally, without distraction. Acceptance, on the other hand, involves an open attitude towards one's experiences, even those that are uncomfortable or unfavorable.

The Harvard Gazette's 2020 report titled "Mind over Body" highlighted the importance of mindfulness in sports by showcasing LeBron James's commitment to mindfulness exercises and the consequential improvement in his game. Players immersed in mindfulness exercises showed improvements in focus, composure under pressure, and recovery from mistakes, demonstrating a significant edge in competitive sports.

8.2. Developing a Mind-Body Training Regimen

To create a regime that better connects the mind and body aspects of training, begin by layering mental exercises into physical team and individual training sessions. Here are some core pillars of a mind-body regimen

1. *Focus Training:* Concentrated focus is integral to any sport. Incorporate exercises that train athletes to concentrate despite distractions. This can be as simple as balancing drills under distracting conditions or more complex exercises like visualization.

2. *Body Awareness:* Body awareness is understanding and feeling the slight changes in balance, posture, and muscle tension needed for precision in movement. Yoga and Taichi are prime examples of activities that can promote greater body awareness.

3. *Emotional Control:* Being able to control the emotional state under pressure is crucial. Mindfulness meditation can be instrumental in achieving emotional control by teaching athletes to observe their emotional state without judgment.

4. *Recovery Rituals:* Adequate rest and recovery are important to the prevention of physical burnout and injuries. Implementing regular periods of relaxation and rejuvenation practices like progressive muscle relaxation can encourage bodily recovery.

8.3. Graduated Integration of Mindfulness

Starting with the basics is the essential first step in developing mindfulness. Every athlete should begin by setting aside specific times each day for mindfulness exercises. These exercises can be as small as a couple of minutes and gradually increase over time.

1. *Mindful Breathing:* This practice involves slowing, regularizing, and focusing solely on one's breath. In stressful or high-pressure situations, mindful breathing can provide an anchor to the present moment.

2. *Guided Imagery:* Guided imagery requires envisioning specific outcomes or actions. For athletes, this could involve visualizing successful execution of a game-winning shot or victory over a challenging opponent.

3. *Body Scan:* The body scan is a progressive process of passing attention across different parts of the body. Regular practice increases awareness of bodily states, facilitating quicker adjustments to balance and precision during athletic performance.

After these basic exercises are a regular part of the athlete's routine, it is then possible to layer higher-level techniques onto their regimen.

8.4. Advanced Techniques

Advanced techniques allow athletes to manipulate their mental state to their advantage.

1. *Flow:* Athletes describe 'flow' as an absorbed state where they lose themselves in the activity leading to stellar performance. Attention training through meditation can guide athletes towards achieving flow states more consistently.

2. *Cognitive Reframe:* This technique involves changing one's perspective towards a stressor. In athletic contexts, reframing an intimidating opponent as a challenge instead of a threat can significantly change an athlete's performance.

3. *Self Talk:* Investigated by researchers as an effective technique to enhance performance, positive self-talk can improve

concentration, effort, and mood. Encouraging athletes to engage in constructive self-dialogue can be a game-changer.

By inculcating such practices, athletes, teams, and coaches can create an environment to harness the power of both mental prowess and physical ability. A harmony of mind-body training paves an effective path for achieving—and sustaining—peak performance. Success, then, becomes more than just a spectator sport and transforms into a synergistic interplay of both mental and physical prowess. The journey towards energetic equipoise is a deep and rewarding one, compelling participants to explore not just the outer, but also the inner workings of their incredible potential.

Chapter 9. The Coach's Role: Fostering Mind-Body Dynamics

The evolution of coaching in sports is a fascinating narrative that speaks to the ever-increasing exhaustive knowledge of the body and its intertwined relationship with the mind. Frequently ensuring command over physical skills and tactics, coaches are now realizing the enormous potential of mental readiness and mindfulness in maximizing performance. Understanding how to cultivate this dynamic interplay becomes a crucial part of the coach's arsenal, empowering athletes to attain an energetic equipoise integral to their success.

9.1. Setting the Stage: Building the Foundation

The first step in fostering mindfulness in athletes centralizes around the coach's role in cultivating a conducive environment for development. The atmosphere should not merely focus on optimizing physical capacity but should equally emphasize nurturing mental growth. A coach's role extends beyond merely imparting technical and tactical knowledge; they stand as a mentor, guide, and confidante, whose impact permeates the often thin divide between personal and professional life of the athletes.

Creating an atmosphere for such holistic growth starts with the recognition that athletes, like everyone else, are unique individuals. Each person approaches the world through a distinctive lens shaped by their experiences, beliefs, and priorities. Attuning to each athlete's personality type and understanding their motivational triggers allow coaches to tailor training protocols and communication styles.

9.2. Cultivating Mindfulness: Strategies in Practice

One of the prime attributes of mindfulness in sports is an athlete's ability to maintain focus during high-pressure moments, often being the difference between a win and a loss. Coaches can incorporate mindfulness techniques into training routines, facilitating increased focus, improved resilience, and better stress management.

Tools such as deep-breathing exercises, progressive muscle relaxation, and visualization techniques are proven effective performance enhancers. For example, short and dedicated periods for silent reflection or meditative practices can be interspersed between physical training sessions. Keeping a training journal to record thoughts, emotions, and reactions during a game or training can also help athletes track their mental growth patterns. Coaches can then review these journals to understand the mental challenges the athletes are going through and guide them accordingly.

9.3. Embracing the Inevitable: Building Resilience Against Failure

In sports, failure is inevitable. However, the power of a coach lies not in avoiding failures for their pupils but in normalizing it and using it as a stepping stone for growth. Emphasizing that failure doesn't diminish their worth as athletes or as people fosters a resilience that's crucial in developing the mental strength required to excel in sports. Coaches can build resilience in athletes by helping them set balanced objectives, concentrating not only on the ultimate goal but also highlighting the value of learning, effort, and personal growth that comes with the journey.

9.4. Encouraging Self-Awareness: Intuition over Instruction

While instruction is a fundamental part of sports, excessive reliance on it can strip athletes of their intuition. Constantly reiterated and often harsh feedback can leave athletes overly fixated on the technical aspects, losing touch with their intuitions and gut feelings about the game. Incorporating specific training blocks where athletes are encouraged to trust their instincts can provide opportunities for developing confidence in their intuitive decision-making, strengthening the mind-body connection.

9.5. Putting it All into Practice: Commitment to Adaptability

Ultimately, to foster energetic equipoise in athletes, coaches need to commit to adaptability. Flexibility in the approach allows for the continuous evolution of athletes as they grow, both physically and mentally. Being open to implement changes in training styles, open to dialogue, and willingness to learn from the athletes themselves underpins the true success of cultivating the mind-body dynamics.

Supplementing physical conditioning with mental training epitomizes the modern-day coach's role. Through the strategic application of mindfulness techniques and practices, coaches can enhance both the mental and physical abilities of athletes. This fusion of the mind and body provides the groundwork for the highest levels of performance, unveiling a new, complete spectrum of potential for athletes to explore.

Fostering this interplay, taking the time to understand each individual, setting realistic and balanced objectives, and being continuously adaptable forms the cornerstone of the coach's role in encouraging mindful, superior sports performance.

Chapter 10. Future Trends: Mindfulness Techniques for Sports Performance

The exploration of mindfulness techniques within sports performance is a rapidly growing field, poised to evolve and expand in the coming years. Notable advancements are on the horizon, predominantly in terms of technique development, applied technology, and scientific research, all converging to optimize an athlete's mental and physical performance.

10.1. Bridging Fields: From Pschychology to Sports Performance

Utilizing mindfulness techniques in sports performance is not a new concept. The foundation lies in the discipline of psychology - where mindfulness techniques were originally developed and honed for therapeutic and wellness purposes. Here, we find emphasis on stress reduction, enhanced communication, cognitive improvement, and an increased ability to manage challenges.

As these concepts spill over into the realm of sports, they bring remarkable enhancements to focus, resilience, flow, and overall performance. Evolving from the traditional imagery, relaxation, and self-talk utilized in sports psychology, mindfulness is a promising addition to an athlete's mental practice regimen. Numerous studies are underway to further explore its impact, particularly in relation to resilience and improved mental health among athletes.

10.2. Applied Technologies: Unleashing the Power of Mindfulness

In an era saturated with digital advancements, integrating technology with mindfulness practices is a logical step toward enhancing sports performance. Apps providing guided meditation, biofeedback devices reporting physiological responses in real-time, VR programmes for immersive mindfulness training - all these technologies are primed to make mindfulness training more accessible, personalised and result-oriented for athletes.

Progress in brain scanning techniques, like fMRI and EEG, is uncovering the neuroscience behind mindfulness, aiding its fine-tuning. Additionally, AI and machine learning play an increasingly pivotal role in analysing biometric data, recommending actions, predicting stressors and evaluating progress in an athlete's mindfulness routine. The intersection of mindfulness and technology holds exciting possibilities for future advancements in sports performance.

10.3. Technique Developments: Evolving Practices for Future Athletes

Mindfulness techniques are branching beyond seated meditation or body scans, leading to a myriad of engaging practices. Mindful movement, for example, is a growing trend. Mindful yoga, martial arts, and mindful walking are all gaining traction in the sports arena. These techniques combine physical training with mental fortitude building, maximizing the benefits of both.

Innovations in the field are also exploring context-specific mindfulness techniques. Tailored mindfulness practices suiting the demands of different sports and their respective competitive environments can better equip athletes in managing sports-related pressures. These bespoke techniques may emerge as game-changers in the sporting world, with early adoption providing athletes a crucial edge.

10.4. The Integral Role of Coaches

Lastly, the role of coaches will evolve alongside these trends. As mindfulness shapes up to be an integral part of performance training, coaches will increasingly need to develop proficiency in incorporating mindfulness strategies into their regimens. Their own mindfulness practices will be necessary to better teach and foster an environment conducive to mindful training. Coach education will have a significant part to play, as institutions and programmes will focus on the amalgamation of sports science with aspects of psychology, neurology, and mindfulness.

As we look towards the future of sports, the application and integration of mindfulness techniques stand on the cusp of major transformations. In a world ever more acknowledging of the balance between physical prowess and mental fortitude for optimal performance, mindfulness will surely be a key player. The metamorphosis will occur not merely within the athletes but also in the systems, the institutions, and the very essence of athletic training, duly redefining the concept of 'energetic equipoise'.

Chapter 11. Maintaining Energetic Equipoise: A Journey, Not A Destination

The axiom of energetic equipoise, that elusive harmony between physical prowess and mental fortitude, gives rise to the ultimate athletic prowess. It's widely recognized, but few have insight into its perceptive mechanisms and practical applications. Drawing deeply on empirical evidence and expert interviews, this detailed discourse will guide you through the journey of maintaining energetic equipoise - a journey, not a destination.

11.1. The Theory of Energetic Equipoise

The most common anecdotal belief around athletic performance centers on physical prowess. Traditional coaching tactics have leaned heavily on strength, speed, and endurance - the tangible aspects of athleticism. However, as the line between top-performing athletes blurs, it's clear these physical factors fail to explain the entire performance.

Energetic equipoise offers an alternate viewpoint. It shifts focus from the tangible to an exciting interplay between physical prowess and mental fortitude. The disparity in the performance of two athletes of similar physical capabilities can often be traced back to their mental conditioning - their resilience, focus, motivation, and based on recent findings, their mindfulness.

This essential mix of physical and mental components is the theory of energetic equipoise. It offers a more holistic view of athleticism that, when applied correctly, can boost an athlete's performance manifold.

11.2. The Role of Mindfulness

Mindfulness, at its core, is an attentive awareness of the reality of things, particularly current happenings. It is being fully immersed, mentally present, and actively engaged in the current activity.

In sports, mindfulness manifests as heightened concentration during training, improved resilience when faced with setbacks, and increased sensitivity towards one's own body. This way, mindfulness optimizes an athlete's 'in-the-moment' decision making, stress management, and ability to avoid or recover from injuries.

One perfect exemplification of mindfulness is seen in legendary tennis player, Novak Djokovic. His attention to not just pure physical training but also mental training like meditation and visualization has solidified his position in the annals of tennis history.

11.3. Implementing Mindfulness Techniques

Now that we've established the theoretical role of mindfulness in energetic equipoise, let's look at concrete ways to bring it into your training regime.

11.3.1. Meditation

Perhaps the most well-known mindfulness technique is meditation. Regular meditation can increase your focus, lower your stress levels, and enhance your resilience. Start with just five minutes a day. Sit in a comfortable position, close your eyes, and focus on the rhythm of your breath. Regularly extend this time as you grow more comfortable with the practice.

11.3.2. Visualization

Next comes visualization, a mental technique that involves picturing the desired outcome in your mind. It allows for better motor control, increases motivation, and can help reduce fear and anxiety. Visualize your moves piece-by-piece in a slow, deliberate fashion. This visualization creates neural patterns in your brain, effectively enhancing muscle memory.

11.3.3. Mindful Eating

Nutrition significantly affects an athlete's performance. Mindful eating involves watching what and how you eat. Consider using a food diary to record your daily consumption. Appreciate each meal and understand the nourishment it offers your body. This approach will amplify the benefits of your dietary regimen while simultaneously promoting healthier eating habits.

These techniques, while simple, require consistent practice. However, the benefits reaped from implementing them far outweigh the requisite commitment.

11.4. The Physical and Mental Balance Through Training

Integrating mindfulness doesn't mean disregarding physical training in any way. However, it requires a refreshed perspective on how both training aspects work cohesively.

Every physical exercise should serve two purposes - strengthening your body and developing your focus. As you engage in strength training, pay attention to the muscles at work. Feel your pulse rising and falling with exertion and rest. Use cardiovascular training to improve not just your endurance, but also your mental resilience.

Moreover, rest, often overlooked, is vital for physical recovery and provides an excellent opportunity for meditation and visualization.

Paying attention to the connections between mind and body augmentation is the first step towards fostering energetic equipoise, aligning your physical prowess with your mental fortitude.

11.5. The Never-Ending Journey

It's crucial to remember that there is no finish line on the track to achieving energetic equipoise. The terrain is always shifting, affected by factors like new research findings, advances in training methods, personal circumstances, and performance metrics.

With this fluidity in mind, athletes should focus on maintaining the balance between their body and mind rather than achieving it. Performance should never plateau. Instead, understanding that physical prowess and mental robustness will require constant cultivation fosters an attitude for continuous growth.

In this vein, energetic equipoise ceases to be an achievement and instead becomes a guiding principle woven into the fabric of an athlete's training regime.

Maintaining Energetic Equipoise: A Journey, Not A Destination, is indeed a never-ending, cyclical process. However, by learning to understand and manipulate its variable aspects - physical prowess, mental fortitude, and mindfulness - we can encourage its positive effect on athletic performance. Embrace this view; embark on your own journey towards a more comprehensive, balanced, and ultimately fruitful athletic experience.